Introduction:

Would you like to reduce stress and feel more calm? Are you looking for a way to be more in touch with the world around you? Do you feel unsure where to start?

This journal is for you!

In just a few minutes each day, you can embark on a new mindfulness journaling practice that can kickstart a new habit, shift your awareness and help you feel more present.

Each day there will be a new prompt and a few questions. Spend 10 minutes (or more) reflecting and writing down your thoughts. This journal is for you and the journey is yours. There are no rules.

You don't need anything special to do these practices and you don't need any prior experience.

Ready to get started? Grab a pen & let's get to it!

I'm so happy that you are here.

Laura

Getting Started:

What are 3 words that describe you?

What apprehensions do you have?

What does mindfulness mean to you?

What is your greatest superpower or strength?

What excites you about this journey?

Day 1:

Find a comfortable place to sit.
Take 3 breaths.
Inhale through the nose and let it out with a sigh.
Let's get started!

A New Lens

Look at something today with fresh, new eyes.
Imagine that this is the first time you've ever seen
it.

This can be anything at all.

A friend, family or loved one. An animal. A scene in
nature. A moment from everyday life.
Really take it all in. Notice it with childlike wonder.

- What do you notice?
- How does it make you feel?
- Does anything come up?
- Are there new details that you may have
  overlooked in the past?
- How does your body feel?

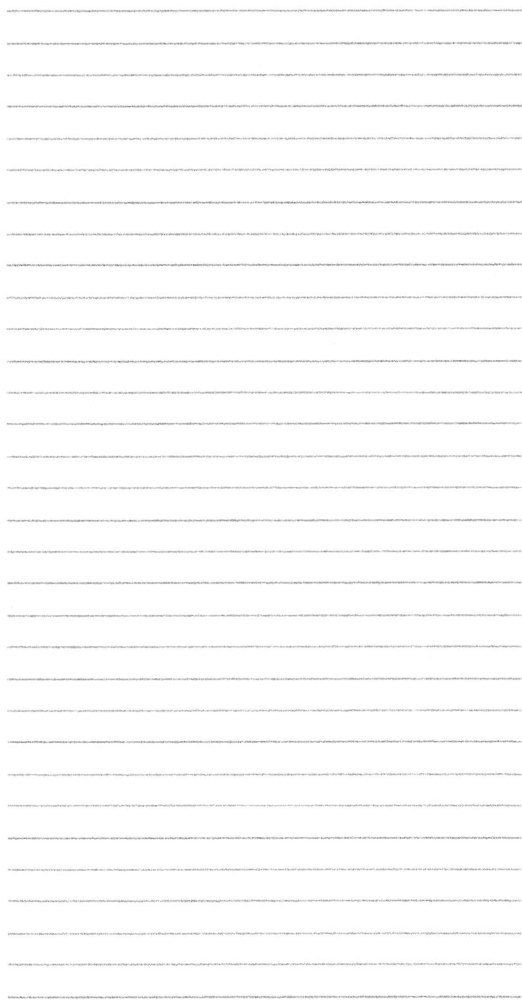

Day 2:

Find a comfortable place to sit.
Take 3 breaths.
Inhale through the nose and let it out with a sigh.
Let's get started!

Senses

Take this time to notice the world through your senses. Look around you.

- What do you see?
    - Note colors, patterns, textures, and shapes.
- What do you hear?
    - Take in sounds near and far.
- What do you smell?
- What do you feel?
- What can you touch?
- Can you taste anything?
- How was this experience?

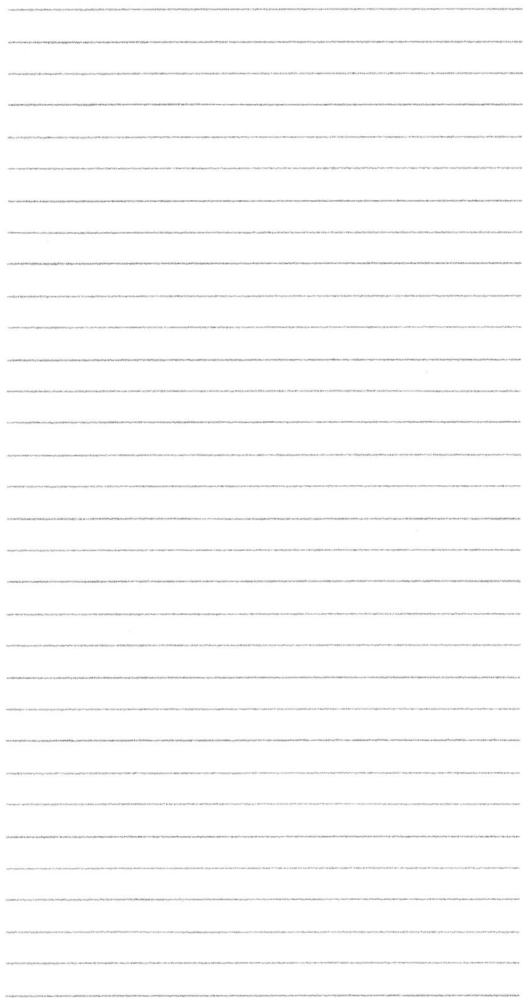

Day 3:

Find a comfortable place to sit.
Take 3 breaths.
Inhale through the nose and let it out with a sigh.
Let's get started!

The Breath

Did you know we take over 20,000 breaths a day?
Today let's tune into our breath.

Be sure you are comfortable, then soften your gaze
or close your eyes.

Where do you feel your breath in your body? What
is its texture? How is its rhythm?

Follow an entire breath cycle from inhale to exhale.

Tune into only your breath. Stay here and notice.

When you are ready, move your body gently and
open your eyes.

- Where did you first feel your breath?
- How did it feel?
- Did it change throughout this exercise?

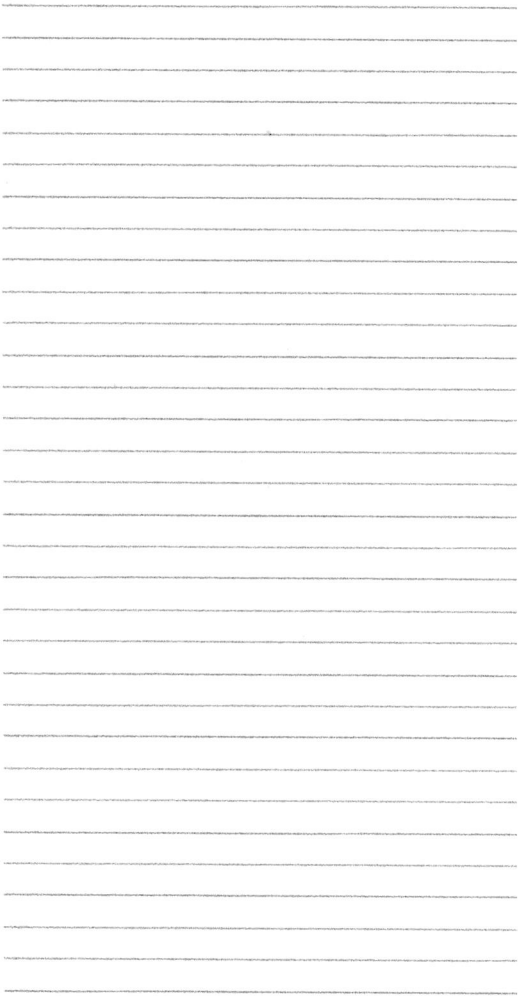

Day 4:

Find a comfortable place to sit.
Take 3 breaths.
Inhale through the nose and let it out with a sigh.
Let's get started!

Body scan

We spend so much time in our minds that we lose touch with our physical body. Today's practice will let you get back in touch, tune in & reconnect with yourself.

Make sure you are comfortably seated or lying down, soften your gaze or close your eyes.
Take a few more relaxed breaths here.

Continue to breathe. Slowly move through the body (Top of the head, forehead, eyes, jaw, tongue, throat, arms, chest, abdomen, pelvis, legs), pausing for several breaths at each stop. Relax and notice. Gently ease back into your breath and body.

- How do you feel after this practice?
- What did you notice?
- Was this practice easy or difficult?

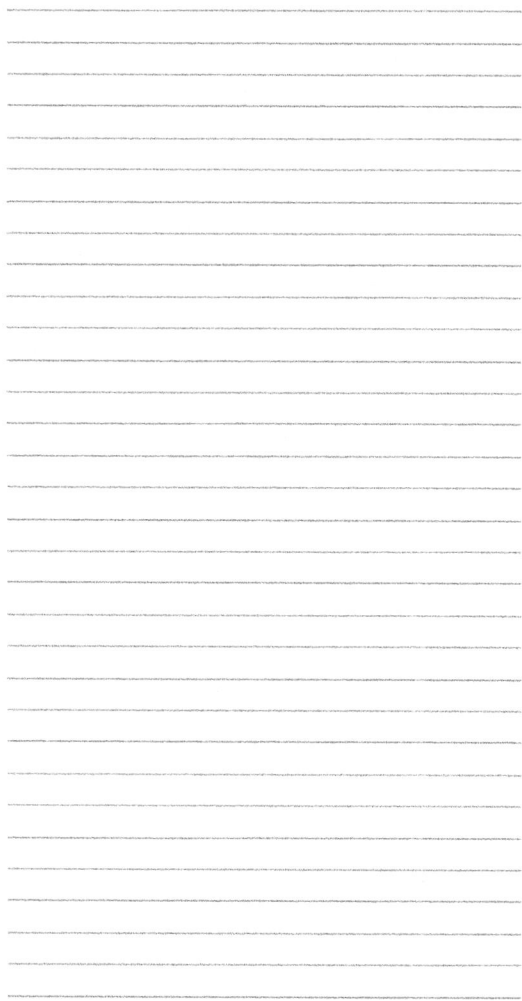

Day 5:

Find a comfortable place to sit.
Take 3 breaths.
Inhale through the nose and let it out with a sigh.
Let's get started!

Mindful Walking

In today's practice we will slow down as we explore the mindfulness of walking. This practice can be done at home, in your office or outside. You just need a small space to walk in a circle or in rows.

Soften your gaze towards the ground and begin to walk slowly. Let the front heel land as you gently move to the ball of the foot and begin to lift the back foot. Continue slowly moving, noticing each area of the foot as it makes contact.

Notice your breath as you move. See if you can slow down your pace even more.

- How did this feel in your body?
- What did you observe?
- How is your mood and energy level?

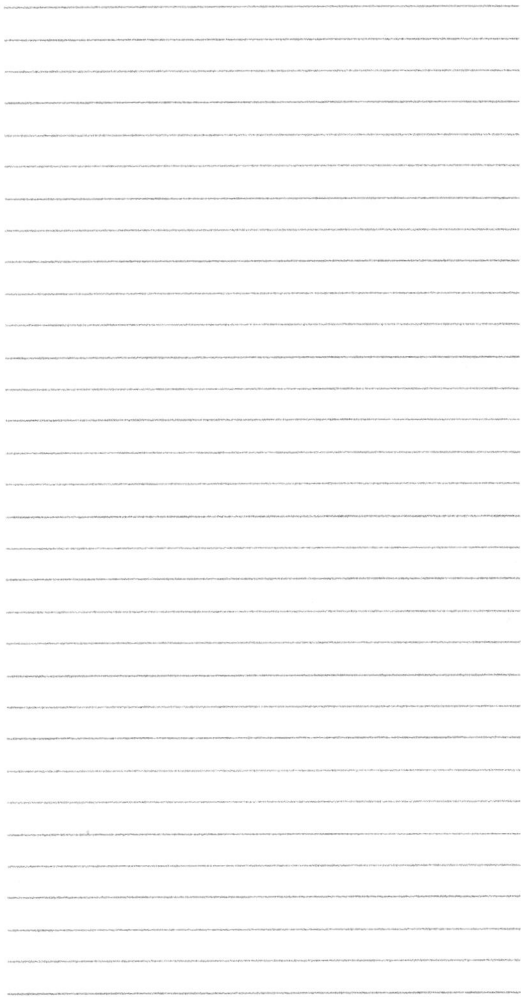

Day 6:

Find a comfortable place to sit.
Take 3 breaths.
Inhale through the nose and let it out with a sigh.
Let's get started!

Coffee or Tea

Grab your favorite beverage and let's begin.

Hold your cup or mug in both hands. Notice the shape and texture. Note the temperature.

Now look inside the cup. Observe the colors. Pay attention to patterns and movement.

Enjoy the aroma and all of the subtleties.

Take a slow sip. Hold it briefly in your mouth before swallowing. Continue drinking at a slow pace.

- What did you notice about this experience?
- How did this differ from drinking without awareness?
- What feelings arose during this practice?
- Did you enjoy this way of drinking?

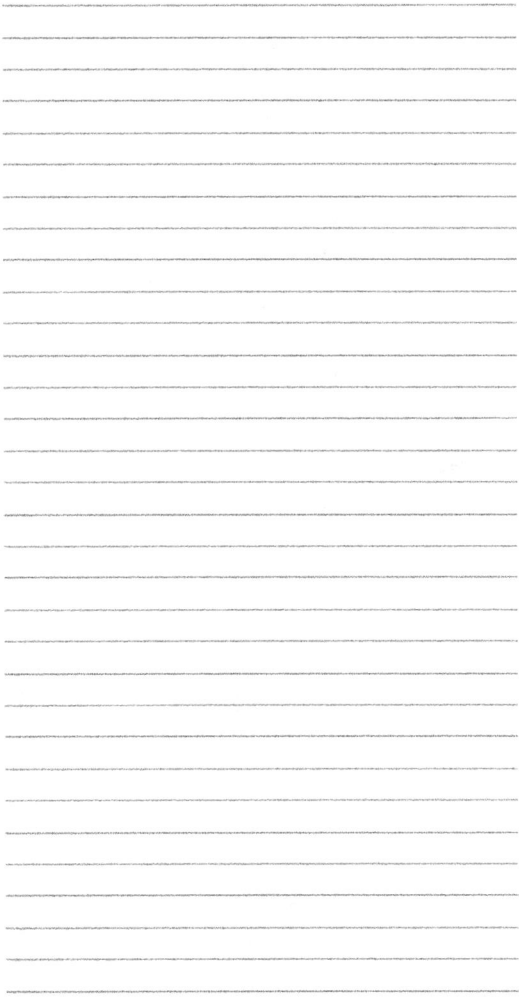

Day 7:

Find a comfortable place to sit.
Take 3 breaths.
Inhale through the nose and let it out with a sigh.
Let's get started!

4:8 Breath

This breath practice can help soothe the nervous system and calm our minds.

Seated or lying down, begin to notice your natural breath.

Fill your lungs on the inhale as you count to 4.
Exhale and empty the lungs as you count to 8.

Try to breathe in and out through the nose. Exhale through your mouth if preferred.

Continue this practice for several cycles then return to your natural breath.

- What did you notice about this practice?
- Did your energy shift?
- How is your mood?
- Were there any challenges?

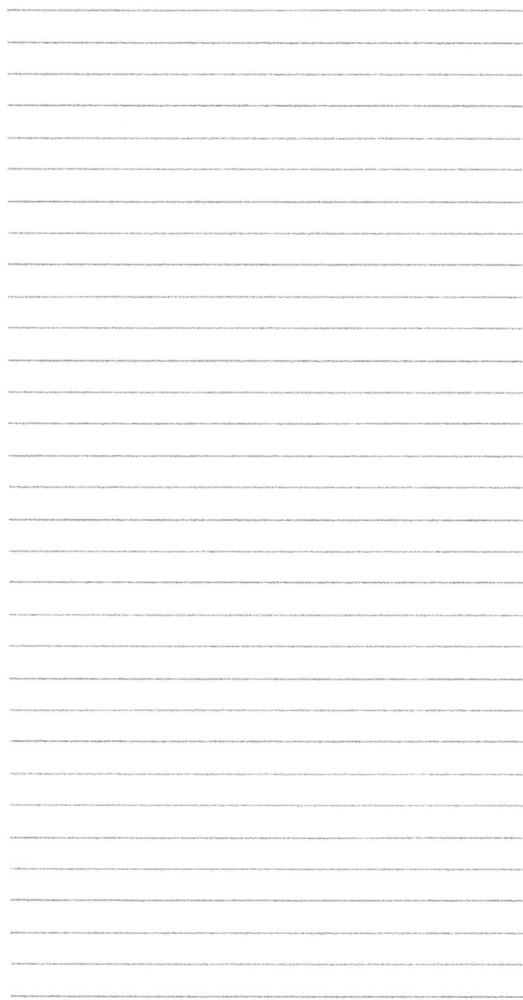

Congratulations!

You've just completed your first week of mindful practices. Be proud of yourself for taking these first steps towards living mindfully.

What was your favorite practice this week?

_____

_____

_____

What was your biggest challenge?

_____

_____

_____

Do you notice any subtle differences?

_____

_____

_____

Did anything special come up?

_____

_____

_____

_____

Thank you for taking this journey.
Want to keep going? Check out Volumes II, III & IV

Additional reflections & thoughts

Additional reflections & thoughts

Additional reflections & thoughts